Forever Young:

A Guide to Living a Healthy and Youthful Life

Passy Campbell

DEDICATION

To those who defy the limits of time,

This book is dedicated to you.

May your journey towards a vibrant and youthful life

Inspire others to embrace the beauty of aging.

TABLE OF CONTENTS

INTRODUCTION

THE CONCEPT OF STAYING FOREVER YOUNG

Welcome to "Forever Young: A Guide to Living a Healthy and Youthful Life." In a world where the pursuit of youthfulness has become a cultural obsession, this book aims to redefine what it means to stay forever young. Rather than chasing an impossible fountain of youth, we will explore a holistic approach to maintaining vitality, well-being, and a youthful mindset throughout our lives.

Aging is a natural process that we all go through, but it doesn't mean we have to accept a decline in our health and vitality. We have the power to influence how we age and the quality of our lives as we grow older. This book will be your comprehensive guide to embracing a lifestyle that promotes health, happiness, and a vibrant existence.

Throughout the chapters of this book, we will dive into various aspects of healthy living. We will explore the science of aging, understanding the factors that contribute to the aging process and how we can slow it down. We will delve into nutrition and diet, discovering the power of food in nourishing our bodies and promoting longevity. We will uncover the importance of exercise and physical activity, finding ways to keep our bodies strong, agile, and full of energy.

Stress management will also be a key topic of discussion, as we explore techniques to cultivate calmness, reduce anxiety, and enhance overall well-being. We will delve into the realm of skincare and beauty, understanding how to care for our skin and maintain a radiant appearance. Mental health and well-being will be another focal point, as we unravel strategies to nurture our minds, boost cognitive function, and find joy in everyday life.

By the end of this book, you will have gained valuable insights and practical tools to incorporate into your daily life. You will have a deeper understanding of how to nourish your body, mind, and soul to stay forever young. Remember, the goal is not to halt the aging process, but to embrace it gracefully while maximizing our potential for happiness, vitality, and longevity.

Get ready to embark on a transformative journey towards a healthier, more youthful version of yourself. Let's embrace the power within us to lead a life that defies age, inspires others, and allows us to truly be forever young.

Why Staying healthy and youthful is important

Staying healthy and youthful is important for several compelling reasons. While aging is a natural process that everyone experiences, taking proactive steps to maintain our health and vitality can greatly enhance our overall well-being and quality of life. Here are some detailed explanations of why staying healthy and youthful is important:

i. **Enhanced Physical Well-being:** Prioritizing our health and adopting a healthy lifestyle can help prevent or manage various chronic diseases and conditions associated with aging. Regular exercise, a balanced diet, and proper nutrition can improve cardiovascular health, maintain healthy weight, strengthen bones and muscles, and boost immune function. By staying healthy, we can minimize the risk of developing conditions such as heart disease, diabetes, osteoporosis, and certain cancers.

ii. Increased Energy and Vitality: Engaging in regular physical activity, eating nutritious foods, and managing stress levels can significantly boost energy levels and overall vitality. When we take care of our bodies and provide them with the necessary nutrients and exercise, we can experience increased stamina, mental alertness, and an overall sense of vigor. This allows us to remain active and fully participate in the activities we enjoy, promoting a fulfilling and active lifestyle.

iii. Mental and Cognitive Benefits: Physical health and mental well-being are interconnected. Research has shown that maintaining a healthy lifestyle can have positive effects on our mental health and cognitive function. Regular exercise releases endorphins, which can alleviate symptoms of depression and anxiety, improve mood, and enhance overall mental well-being. Additionally, a balanced diet rich in nutrients supports brain health and can help prevent cognitive decline, promoting sharper memory, better focus, and improved cognitive abilities as we age.

iv. Improved Emotional Well-being: Taking care of our physical health also has a profound impact on our emotional well-being. When we feel physically fit and healthy, it can boost self-esteem and self-confidence, leading to a more positive body image and increased overall happiness. Engaging in stress management techniques, such as mindfulness and relaxation practices, can reduce anxiety, promote emotional resilience, and enhance our ability to cope with the challenges of life.

v. Longevity and Quality of Life: By adopting a healthy lifestyle, we can potentially increase our lifespan and enjoy a higher quality of life as we age. When we prioritize our health and well-being, we are more likely to maintain independence, engage in fulfilling relationships and activities, and experience a greater sense of fulfillment and purpose. Staying healthy allows us to make the most of our years and enjoy a vibrant and active life well into old age.

In summary, staying healthy and youthful is important because it enhances physical well-being, boosts energy and vitality, improves mental and cognitive function, enhances emotional well-being, and promotes longevity and a higher quality of life. By taking proactive steps to prioritize our health, we can experience the fullness of life and age gracefully while enjoying the benefits of a vibrant and

youthful existence.

CHAPTER ONE

THE SCIENCE OF AGING

"The Science of Aging" is a fascinating field of study that explores the processes

and factors that contribute to the aging of the human body. It encompasses

various biological, genetic, and environmental factors that influence how we age.

Understanding the science behind aging is crucial for developing effective

strategies to slow down the aging process and promote healthy longevity.

How the body ages

Aging involves a complex interplay of biological processes that occur at the cellular, molecular, and systemic levels. Over time, our cells undergo cumulative damage and experience a decline in their functional abilities. This is primarily attributed to a gradual loss of cellular integrity, DNA damage, telomere shortening, and impaired protein function. These processes lead to a gradual decline in organ function, reduced tissue repair and regeneration, and increased vulnerability to diseases.

The role of genetics in aging

Genetics plays a significant role in determining how we age. Certain genetic variations and predispositions can influence the rate at which our body ages. For instance, variations in genes responsible for DNA repair mechanisms, telomere maintenance, inflammation regulation, and oxidative stress response can impact the aging process. However, it's important to note that while genetics sets the foundation, lifestyle and environmental factors can modulate how these genetic factors are expressed.

The impact of lifestyle factors on aging

While genetics sets the stage, lifestyle factors play a crucial role in shaping the aging process. Unhealthy lifestyle habits, such as poor nutrition, sedentary behavior, chronic stress, inadequate sleep, and exposure to toxins, can accelerate the aging process. Conversely, adopting a healthy lifestyle that includes a balanced diet, regular physical activity, stress management techniques, sufficient sleep, and avoidance of harmful substances can help slow down the aging process and promote longevity.

Introduction to anti-aging strategies

Anti-aging strategies aim to counteract the effects of aging and promote healthy aging. These strategies encompass a range of approaches, including lifestyle modifications, dietary interventions, skincare practices, and the use of specific anti-aging treatments. Lifestyle modifications focus on maintaining a healthy weight, engaging in regular exercise, managing stress, and avoiding harmful habits like smoking and excessive alcohol consumption. A nutrient-rich diet, including antioxidants, anti-inflammatory foods, and adequate hydration, can support cellular health and combat age-related damage. Skincare practices involve protecting the skin from sun damage, using moisturizers and targeted products, and incorporating healthy habits like proper cleansing and adequate hydration.

Additionally, emerging anti-aging treatments and therapies, such as hormone replacement therapy, stem cell therapies, and certain pharmaceutical interventions, are being explored.

In conclusion, the science of aging encompasses the understanding of how the body ages, the influence of genetics, the impact of lifestyle factors, and the introduction to anti-aging strategies. By comprehending these aspects, we can make informed choices to promote healthy aging and implement strategies to slow down the aging process, maintain vitality, and enhance our overall well-being as we grow older.

CHAPTER TWO

NUTRITION AND DIET

Nutrition and diet play a crucial role in the aging process, affecting our overall health, well-being, and longevity. This chapter explores the importance of nutrition in aging, highlights the best foods for anti-aging, discusses common dietary pitfalls, and provides practical tips for healthy eating and meal planning.

The role of nutrition in aging

Nutrition plays a fundamental role in supporting cellular health, maintaining organ function, and preventing age-related diseases. As we age, our body's nutrient requirements may change, and certain nutrients become even more important. Adequate intake of essential vitamins, minerals, antioxidants, and phytochemicals can help protect against oxidative stress, inflammation, and cellular damage. Proper nutrition also supports healthy immune function, bone density, and cognitive function, promoting optimal aging.

The best foods for anti-aging

Certain foods have been recognized for their anti-aging properties and ability to support health as we age. These include:

1. Fruits and vegetables: Colorful fruits and vegetables are rich in antioxidants, vitamins, and minerals. Berries, leafy greens, citrus fruits, and cruciferous vegetables are particularly beneficial due to their high content of vitamins C, E, and A, as well as phytochemicals that combat cellular damage and inflammation.

2. Healthy fats: Omega-3 fatty acids found in fatty fish (such as salmon and sardines), flaxseeds, and walnuts provide anti-inflammatory benefits and support brain health. Monounsaturated fats from olive oil, avocados, and nuts can help protect against heart disease.

3. Whole grains: High-fiber whole grains like quinoa, brown rice, and oats provide sustained energy and support digestive health. They also contain essential nutrients and phytochemicals that contribute to overall well-being.

4. Lean proteins: Opt for lean protein sources such as poultry, fish, beans, lentils, and tofu. These provide essential amino acids for muscle repair, immune function, and hormone production.

Common dietary pitfalls and how to avoid them

Common dietary pitfalls include excessive consumption of processed foods, sugary snacks, unhealthy fats, and sodium. These can contribute to inflammation, weight gain, and chronic diseases. To avoid these pitfalls, it is important to prioritize whole, minimally processed foods. Limit added sugars, unhealthy fats (such as trans fats and saturated fats), and high-sodium foods. Instead, focus on nutrient-dense options and be mindful of portion sizes.

Tips for healthy eating and meal planning:

1. Eat a balanced diet: Include a variety of fruits, vegetables, whole grains, lean proteins, and healthy fats in your meals to ensure you get a wide range of nutrients.

2. Portion control: Be mindful of portion sizes to maintain a healthy weight and prevent overeating. Use smaller plates and bowls to control portions visually.

3. Meal planning: Plan your meals in advance to ensure a balanced and nutritious diet. This helps avoid impulsive food choices and promotes healthier eating habits.

4. Hydration: Stay adequately hydrated by drinking plenty of water throughout the day. Limit sugary beverages and alcohol.

5. Mindful eating: Practice mindful eating by slowing down, savoring your meals, and paying attention to hunger and fullness cues.

6. Seek professional guidance: Consult a registered dietitian or nutritionist who can provide personalized recommendations based on your specific needs and health goals.

By understanding the role of nutrition in aging, incorporating anti-aging foods into our diet, avoiding common dietary pitfalls, and implementing healthy eating practices, we can nourish our bodies, support optimal aging, and promote long-term health and vitality.

CHAPTER THREE

EXERCISE AND PHYSICAL ACTIVITY

Exercise and physical activity are essential components of a healthy and youthful lifestyle. This chapter explores the importance of exercise for anti-aging, provides an overview of the best types of exercise for staying young, offers tips for incorporating exercise into your daily routine, and emphasizes the significance of strength training and flexibility exercises.

The importance of exercise for anti-aging

Regular exercise has numerous benefits for both physical and mental well-being, making it a powerful tool for anti-aging. Exercise helps improve cardiovascular health, maintain a healthy weight, enhance muscle strength and tone, increase bone density, and improve balance and coordination. It also promotes healthy brain function, reduces the risk of chronic diseases, boosts immune function, and enhances overall quality of life. Engaging in regular exercise can help slow down the aging process, improve longevity, and increase vitality.

The best types of exercise for staying young

1. Aerobic Exercise: Activities such as brisk walking, jogging, swimming, cycling, and dancing increase heart rate, improve cardiovascular health, and enhance endurance. Aim for at least 150 minutes of moderate-intensity aerobic exercise or 75 minutes of vigorous-intensity exercise per week.

2. Strength Training: Incorporate resistance training exercises to build and maintain muscle strength. This can include weightlifting, bodyweight exercises, or the use of resistance bands. Aim for two or more days of strength training per week, targeting major muscle groups.

3. Flexibility and Balance Exercises: Stretching exercises and activities like yoga, Pilates, and tai chi improve flexibility, balance, and posture. These exercises promote joint mobility, reduce the risk of falls, and help maintain an active lifestyle.

4. Functional Training: Incorporate exercises that mimic everyday movements to improve overall functionality and prevent age-related declines in physical abilities. This can include exercises like squats, lunges, and core-strengthening exercises.

Tips for incorporating exercise Into your daily routine

1. Start slowly and progress gradually: If you're new to exercise, start with low-impact activities and gradually increase intensity and duration over time. Listen to your body and avoid overexertion.

2. Find activities you enjoy: Choose exercises that you find enjoyable and that suit your interests and fitness level. This increases the likelihood of sticking with a regular exercise routine.

3. Make it a habit: Schedule exercise into your daily routine, treating it as a non-negotiable appointment. Consistency is key for long-term benefits.

4. Break it up: If finding a block of time for exercise is challenging, break it up into smaller sessions throughout the day. For example, take a brisk walk during your lunch break or engage in short exercise routines at home.

5. Stay motivated: Set goals, track your progress, and reward yourself for achieving milestones. Exercise with a friend or join group classes for added motivation and accountability.

The importance of strength training and flexibility exercises

Strength training exercises help maintain muscle mass, improve metabolism, and preserve bone density, which can decline with age. Building and maintaining muscle strength is crucial for mobility, balance, and overall functionality. Flexibility exercises, on the other hand, promote joint health, improve range of motion, and reduce the risk of injuries. Incorporating both strength training and flexibility exercises into your exercise routine can contribute to a well-rounded fitness regimen and support healthy aging.

In conclusion, regular exercise and physical activity are vital for anti-aging. Engaging in aerobic exercise, strength training, flexibility exercises, and functional training can help improve cardiovascular health, muscle strength, flexibility, balance, and overall well-being. By incorporating exercise into your daily routine, starting gradually, and finding activities you enjoy, you can experience the numerous benefits of exercise and promote a healthy and youthful lifestyle.

CHAPTER FOUR

STRESS MANAGEMENT

Stress is an inevitable part of life, but how we manage it can significantly impact our overall well-being and the aging process. This chapter delves into the impact of stress on aging, provides practical tips for managing stress and anxiety, explores relaxation techniques like meditation and yoga, and emphasizes the importance of self-care.

The impact of stress on aging

Chronic stress can have detrimental effects on both our physical and mental health, contributing to accelerated aging. Prolonged exposure to stress hormones like cortisol can disrupt the body's natural balance, leading to increased inflammation, impaired immune function, and damage to cells and tissues. Over time, this can contribute to the development of chronic diseases, such as cardiovascular conditions, diabetes, and mental health disorders. Additionally, stress can manifest as unhealthy coping mechanisms like emotional eating, lack of exercise, poor sleep, and substance abuse, all of which can further exacerbate the aging process.

Tips for managing stress and anxiety

1. Identify stress triggers: Recognize the situations, people, or activities that tend to cause stress in your life. By identifying triggers, you can take proactive steps to minimize their impact or develop strategies to cope effectively.

2. Practice time management: Prioritize tasks, set realistic goals, and establish boundaries to reduce overwhelm and create a sense of control over your schedule. Effective time management can help alleviate stress and create a more balanced lifestyle.

3. Develop healthy coping mechanisms: Instead of turning to unhealthy habits, cultivate positive coping mechanisms to manage stress. Engage in activities like exercise, hobbies, journaling, or spending time in nature to help alleviate stress and promote relaxation.

4. Seek support: Reach out to friends, family, or professionals for support and guidance. Sharing your concerns and seeking advice can provide emotional relief and new perspectives.

Overview of relaxation techniques, such as meditation and yoga

Meditation and yoga are powerful relaxation techniques that can help reduce stress and promote a sense of calm and well-being.

Meditation:

Meditation is a practice that involves training the mind to focus and redirect thoughts, leading to a state of clarity and calmness. It is often used as a tool for stress management due to its ability to promote relaxation and reduce anxiety. During meditation, individuals typically sit or lie down in a comfortable position, close their eyes, and engage in techniques such as deep breathing, mindfulness, or visualization. By intentionally directing attention to the present moment and letting go of distracting thoughts, meditation helps to quiet the mind, alleviate stress, and cultivate a sense of inner peace. Regular practice can lead to increased self-awareness, improved emotional well-being, and better resilience in dealing with everyday stressors.

Yoga:

Yoga is a holistic practice originating from ancient India that integrates physical postures, breathing exercises, meditation, and ethical principles. It combines physical movement, breath control, and mental focus to promote physical strength, flexibility, balance, and mental well-being. As a stress management tool, yoga offers a multidimensional approach. The physical postures, known as asanas, help release physical tension and improve circulation, which can have a positive impact on reducing stress levels. The breathing exercises, known as pranayama, help regulate the breath and activate the body's relaxation response, promoting a sense of calmness. Additionally, yoga incorporates mindfulness and meditation techniques, enhancing mental clarity and reducing stress-related thoughts. Regular practice of yoga can contribute to better stress management by cultivating a harmonious connection between the body, mind, and spirit, leading to overall well-being

The importance of self-care

Self-care is essential for maintaining overall well-being and managing stress. It involves engaging in activities that nourish and rejuvenate the body, mind, and soul. Self-care practices can vary from person to person but may include activities like practicing mindfulness, taking time for hobbies and interests, engaging in relaxation exercises, getting sufficient sleep, and nurturing social connections. Prioritizing self-care allows us to recharge, reduce stress levels, and enhance our ability to cope with life's challenges.

Summarily, effective stress management is crucial for healthy aging. By understanding the impact of stress on the aging process, adopting strategies to manage stress and anxiety, incorporating relaxation techniques like meditation and yoga, and prioritizing self-care, we can reduce the negative effects of stress and promote overall well-being. Taking proactive steps to manage stress contributes to a more youthful and vibrant life, both mentally and physically.

CHAPTER FIVE

Skincare plays a significant role in the aging process, as it directly impacts the health and appearance of our skin. In this chapter, let's discuss the impact of skincare on aging, an overview of the best skincare practices for staying youthful, common skincare concerns such as wrinkles and sun damage, and also tips for natural beauty treatments and anti-aging products.

The impact of skincare on aging

Skincare is essential for maintaining healthy, youthful-looking skin and combating the signs of aging. As we age, our skin undergoes various changes, including a decline in collagen and elastin production, decreased skin cell turnover, and increased vulnerability to environmental damage. Skincare practices can help nourish and protect the skin, improve its texture and tone, and minimize the appearance of fine lines, wrinkles, and other age-related concerns. Consistent skincare routines can enhance skin health, boost confidence, and contribute to a more youthful appearance.

Overview of the best skincare practices for staying youthful

1. Cleansing: Proper cleansing is the foundation of a good skincare routine. Use a gentle cleanser to remove impurities, dirt, and excess oil without stripping the skin of its natural moisture.

2. Moisturizing: Hydration is key to maintaining youthful skin. Choose a moisturizer suited to your skin type to replenish moisture, improve elasticity, and create a protective barrier against external aggressors.

3. Sun Protection: Protecting your skin from harmful UV rays is crucial for preventing premature aging. Apply a broad-spectrum sunscreen with an SPF of 30 or higher daily, and seek shade during peak sun hours.

4. Exfoliation: Regular exfoliation removes dead skin cells, promotes cell turnover, and reveals fresh, radiant skin. Use chemical exfoliants or gentle physical exfoliators suited to your skin type.

5. Anti-Aging Ingredients: Incorporate skincare products with anti-aging ingredients such as retinol, vitamin C, peptides, and hyaluronic acid. These ingredients can help reduce the appearance of wrinkles, improve skin texture, and enhance overall skin health.

Common skincare concerns, such as wrinkles and sun damage

1. Wrinkles: Wrinkles are a common sign of aging. To address wrinkles, use products with ingredients like retinol, which can stimulate collagen production and promote skin renewal. Consider incorporating targeted treatments, such as eye creams or serums, for specific areas prone to wrinkles.

2. Sun Damage: Prolonged sun exposure contributes to skin aging and increases the risk of skin cancer. Apart from using sunscreen, consider products with antioxidants like vitamin C and green tea extract to protect against free radicals caused by sun damage.

Tips for natural beauty treatments and anti-aging products

1. Natural Beauty Treatments: Incorporate natural remedies like DIY facial masks using ingredients like honey, yogurt, and avocado, which can hydrate, nourish, and brighten the skin. Additionally, natural oils like rosehip oil and argan oil can provide hydration and antioxidants.

2. Anti-Aging Products: Look for anti-aging products that are formulated with scientifically proven ingredients and have positive customer reviews. Consider seeking advice from dermatologists or skincare professionals to find products that are suitable for your skin type and concerns.

3. Lifestyle Factors: Remember that skincare is not just about products; lifestyle factors also play a role. Prioritize a healthy diet, hydration, regular exercise, stress management, and sufficient sleep to support overall skin health.

Effective skincare practices are essential for maintaining youthful, healthy-looking skin which can be achieved by understanding the impact of skincare on aging, adopting a comprehensive skincare routine that includes cleansing, moisturizing, sun protection, exfoliation, and the use of anti-aging ingredients, addressing common skincare concerns, and incorporating natural beauty.

CHAPTER SIX

MENTAL HEALTH AND WELL-BEING

Mental health and well-being are fundamental aspects of living a healthy and youthful life. This chapter explores the importance of mental health for anti-aging, discusses common mental health concerns such as depression and anxiety, provides an overview of natural remedies and treatments for mental health, and offers tips for staying mentally sharp and engaged.

The importance of mental health for anti-aging

Mental health plays a crucial role in overall well-being and has a direct impact on the aging process. Our mental state influences how we perceive and cope with stress, maintain relationships, make decisions, and engage in self-care practices. Neglecting mental health can lead to increased levels of stress, emotional imbalance, and impaired cognitive function, which can contribute to accelerated aging. Conversely, prioritizing mental health promotes resilience, emotional stability, and cognitive vitality, fostering a more youthful and vibrant outlook on life.

Common mental health concerns

Depression: Depression is a prevalent mental health condition that can negatively impact quality of life and overall well-being. It is characterized by persistent sadness, loss of interest in activities, changes in appetite or sleep patterns, and feelings of hopelessness. Seeking professional help and engaging in therapeutic interventions can effectively address and manage depression.

Anxiety: Anxiety disorders involve excessive worry, fear, and unease, which can interfere with daily functioning. Anxiety can manifest in various forms, such as generalized anxiety disorder, panic disorder, or social anxiety disorder. Effective treatment options include therapy, medication, and lifestyle changes.

Natural remedies and treatments for mental health

1. Mindfulness and Meditation: Practicing mindfulness and meditation can help calm the mind, reduce stress, and promote emotional well-being. These techniques involve focusing attention on the present moment, cultivating self-awareness, and developing a non-judgmental attitude towards thoughts and feelings.

2. Exercise: Physical activity is not only beneficial for physical health but also has a positive impact on mental well-being. Regular exercise releases endorphins, which are natural mood-boosting chemicals. Engaging in activities like walking, yoga, or dancing can enhance mood, reduce anxiety, and improve overall mental health.

3. Social Support: Maintaining healthy social connections and seeking support from friends, family, or support groups can provide emotional relief, foster a sense of belonging, and mitigate feelings of loneliness or isolation.

4. Sleep: Prioritizing quality sleep is essential for mental health. Establishing a consistent sleep routine, creating a comfortable sleep environment, and practicing relaxation techniques before bed can improve sleep quality and support overall mental well-being.

Tips for staying mentally sharp and engaged

1. Lifelong Learning: Engage in continuous learning and intellectual stimulation to keep the mind active and sharp. Read books, take up new hobbies, solve puzzles, or participate in educational courses or workshops.

2. Social and Emotional Engagement: Cultivate meaningful relationships, engage in social activities, and express emotions openly. Connecting with others and expressing emotions can contribute to a sense of purpose, happiness, and overall mental well-being.

3. Stress Management: Adopt stress management techniques such as deep breathing exercises, journaling, or engaging in activities that promote relaxation. Effective stress management helps maintain mental resilience and reduces the risk of mental health issues.

4. Self-Care: Prioritize self-care activities that nourish your mind, body, and soul. Engage in activities that bring you joy, practice self-compassion, and set boundaries to protect your mental well-being.

Prioritizing mental health and well-being is essential for a healthy and youthful life. By understanding the importance of mental health, addressing common mental health concerns, incorporating natural remedies and treatments, and adopting tips for staying mentally sharp and engaged, we can promote emotional well-being, enhance cognitive vitality, and cultivate a positive mindset that contributes to overall anti-aging efforts.

CHAPTER SEVEN

THE ANTI-AGING LIFESTYLE

Bringing it all together, the anti-aging lifestyle; in the previous chapters, we have explored various aspects of living a healthy and youthful life. Now, it's time to bring all the strategies and practices together into a comprehensive anti-aging lifestyle. By incorporating these strategies into your daily life, you can maximize their benefits and promote long-term well-being.

Tips for incorporating all of the strategies discussed into your life

1. Create a Routine: Establish a daily routine that includes time for exercise, healthy eating, skincare, stress management, and mental well-being. Set specific goals and allocate dedicated time for each aspect of the anti-aging lifestyle.

2. Start Small: Implementing all of the strategies at once can be overwhelming. Begin by focusing on one or two areas that resonate with you the most and gradually incorporate additional practices over time. Remember, small, consistent steps lead to lasting changes.

3. Accountability and Support: Seek support from family, friends, or online communities to stay motivated and accountable. Share your goals and progress, and celebrate achievements together. Having a support system can provide encouragement and help you stay on track.

4. Track Your Progress: Keep a journal or use an app to track your progress and document the positive changes you experience. This can serve as a reminder of the benefits and motivate you to continue embracing the anti-aging lifestyle.

The benefits of staying forever young include:

1. Enhanced Physical Health: By following the anti-aging lifestyle, you can experience improved physical health. Regular exercise strengthens muscles and bones, boosts cardiovascular health, and increases energy levels. A nutritious diet can reduce the risk of chronic diseases and provide essential nutrients for overall well-being.

2. Youthful Appearance: Skincare practices and healthy habits can contribute to a radiant, youthful complexion. Protecting your skin from sun damage, incorporating anti-aging ingredients, and following a consistent skincare routine can minimize the appearance of wrinkles, fine lines, and age spots.

3. Mental Well-Being: Prioritizing mental health and well-being can lead to increased resilience, improved cognitive function, and reduced risk of mental health disorders. By managing stress, practicing relaxation techniques, and engaging in activities that bring joy and fulfillment, you can maintain a positive outlook and enjoy a youthful mindset.

4. Quality of Life: The anti-aging lifestyle promotes overall quality of life. By embracing healthy habits, you can experience increased vitality, improved mood, and a greater sense of fulfillment. These factors contribute to a more vibrant and fulfilling life at any age.

Final thoughts and encouragement

Embracing the anti-aging lifestyle is a journey that requires commitment, perseverance, and self-care. Remember that every positive step you take towards a healthier and more youthful life matters. Be patient with yourself, as lasting changes take time.

Incorporate the strategies discussed in this book into your daily life gradually, customizing them to fit your unique needs and preferences. Stay mindful of the importance of nutrition, exercise, stress management, skincare, and mental well-being. Embrace self-care and prioritize activities that bring joy, fulfillment, and relaxation.

You have the power to shape your own aging process. By adopting the anti-aging lifestyle, you are taking control of your health and well-being, setting the stage for a vibrant and youthful future. Embrace the journey with confidence, knowing that each step you take brings you closer to living a healthier, happier, and more youthful life.

Remember! Age is just a number, and you have the ability to stay forever young in spirit, mind, and body.

CONCLUSION

In "Forever Young: A Guide to Living a Healthy and Youthful Life," we have delved into the essential elements of maintaining a vibrant and youthful lifestyle. From understanding the science of aging to incorporating nutrition, exercise, stress management, skincare, and mental well-being practices, we have explored a holistic approach to anti-aging. As we conclude this book, let us recap the main points and strategies discussed, while encouraging you to embark on your own journey towards a healthier, happier, and more youthful life.

Throughout this book, we have emphasized the importance of taking charge of your health and well-being. We have explored how the body ages and the role of genetics in the aging process. We have learned how lifestyle factors, such as nutrition, exercise, stress management, skincare, and mental well-being, can significantly impact the aging process and overall vitality.

By focusing on nutrition and incorporating a balanced diet rich in anti-aging foods, we provide our bodies with the essential nutrients and antioxidants needed for optimal health and youthful vitality. We have also discussed common dietary pitfalls and offered tips for healthy eating and meal planning, empowering you to make informed choices.

Furthermore, we have emphasized the significance of exercise in the anti-aging journey. Regular physical activity not only helps maintain a healthy weight and cardiovascular fitness but also promotes strength, flexibility, and overall well-being. We have highlighted the best types of exercises for staying young and provided practical tips for incorporating exercise into your daily routine. Additionally, we have stressed the importance of strength training and flexibility exercises, as they play a vital role in preserving muscle mass, bone density, and mobility.

Stress management has emerged as a crucial aspect of maintaining a youthful and healthy life. By recognizing the impact of stress on aging, we have explored various strategies for managing stress and anxiety. From mindfulness and meditation to relaxation techniques like yoga, we have provided tools for cultivating calm and finding inner peace. We have also discussed the importance of self-care and the role it plays in nurturing our mental, emotional, and physical well-being.

Skincare has been shown to have a significant impact on the aging process. We have examined the best skincare practices for maintaining a youthful appearance and addressing common concerns such as wrinkles and sun damage. By adopting a consistent skincare routine, protecting our skin from harmful UV rays, and incorporating natural beauty treatments and anti-aging products, we can enhance our skin's health and radiance.

Mental health and well-being are foundational pillars of a youthful lifestyle. By acknowledging the importance of mental health and addressing common concerns like depression and anxiety, we have explored natural remedies and treatments to support emotional well-being. We have encouraged lifelong learning, social engagement, and stress management techniques as ways to nurture our minds and maintain cognitive vitality.

In conclusion, we urge you to embrace the knowledge and strategies shared in this book and take the necessary steps to live a healthy and youthful life. Remember that it is never too late to start on the path to rejuvenation and well-being. Your health and vitality are within your control, and every positive choice you make contributes to a more vibrant and fulfilling life.

We encourage you to prioritize your health, make conscious decisions about your nutrition and exercise, manage stress effectively, invest in self-care, and foster a positive mindset. Embrace the anti-aging lifestyle with enthusiasm, knowing that you have the power to shape your own aging journey.

Now is the time to take action and embark on this transformative journey towards a healthier, happier, and more youthful you. Start today and embrace the incredible benefits that await you. You have the ability to live a life that defies age and radiates vitality. Embrace the challenge, believe in your potential, and let your journey to a healthy and youthful life begin.